AJAY'S JOURNEY

FROM SETBACK TO STRENGTH WITH HIS OWN PERSEVERANCE METHODS

By

Ajay Patel

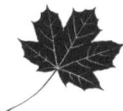

MAPLE
PUBLISHERS

Ajay's Journey from Setback to Strength with his own Perseverance Methods

Author: Ajay Patel

Copyright © Ajay Patel (2025)

The right of Ajay Patel to be identified as author of this work has been asserted by the author in accordance with section 77 and 78 of the Copyright, Designs and Patents Act 1988.

First Published in 2025

ISBN 978-1-83538-666-8 (Paperback)
 978-1-83538-667-5 (Hardback)
 978-1-83538-668-2 (E-Book)

Book cover design and Book layout by:
 White Magic Studios
 www.whitemagicstudios.co.uk

Published by:
 Maple Publishers
 Fairbourne Drive, Atterbury,
 Milton Keynes,
 MK10 9RG, UK
 www.maplepublishers.com

Dedication

This book is dedicated to Amit, Asit, Roma, Anisha (MD) and Shreya (CEO) - without whom I would not be here. Their support, inspiration and guidance has saved me.

Also, a special mention to Nishil, Krishan and Kinnari (my children), Ramesh Uncle, lla Aunty, Krishan, Tony, Simon O'Leary, Avtar Baines, Nagin Kaka's family (Neelima, Talika) and Mukta Aunty (she always sends me my favourite snacks that my mum taught her to make. I love that because I love the memories of my mother).

I would also like to thank Suresh and Joshana, Sai Kommu, Raghu, Ash and Anny from Autumn Care.

Thank you all for your unwavering support and inspiration throughout this journey from a severe stroke to recovery and success in life. Together, you have helped me on my road to recovery and made this book possible.

Contents

Chapter 1
Early Years

To start at the beginning, my parents were from India and had a very traditional Indian wedding. They were married at 16 - the typical age that people married in those days. It was the year 1934.

When the British left India in 1947, they selected skilled people to help in the development of services in East Africa. Dad was a dermatologist, and his father had been an accountant. The family decided they would go to East Africa and make their mark there. The British helped them to move. Initially, they were based in Kampala, but Dad found he couldn't get work. Eventually, however, he got a job in North Uganda in Gulu where he made a very good circle of friends. He loved playing volleyball and cricket. Those friends he made are still in touch, calling often to see if we are OK. They were more like family than friends. My three brothers and I were all born in East Africa, quite late in my parents' lives.

I was the last child, and I was born on the 28th of March 1968. My parents had travelled from Kampala to Arusha, Tanzania for a family wedding, and I made an earlier than expected appearance, in a hospital in Arusha.

My father was eventually offered a very good job in Kampala.

We lived happily in Kampala until Idi Amin decided to kick all the Asians out of the country, 200,000 men women and children.

The hidden rumour behind it was that Idi Amin had fallen in love with an Indian woman who had refused him. However, it is certainly true that he also thought that the Asians in Uganda were taking over the economy of the country.

We had to leave everything behind us and flee. Dad had been given the heads up through people he worked with. My three brothers were sent to boarding school in India and Mum, and I travelled to Gujarat for a couple of years, a time that was really difficult for Mum. She had a lot to worry about. We lived with my cousin and my cousin's sister visited every week. Her name was Malti ben, and I was so thrilled when she came, as she took me out for ice cream and quite often to see a movie. It was the highlight of my week. Malti-ben would keep me on top of things study-wise too. Mum always wanted a daughter but had us four boys. She said to Malti-ben once that she wanted her to be her daughter. They loved each other a lot and were inseparable.

Dad left Uganda with minimum money in his pocket. He had a love of Persian carpets, and he had bought many. All had to be left behind. He left with only the clothes on his back.

On the way to the airport, cars were stopped, and the Asian ladies were dragged out and told to hand over their jewellery. It was an experience that was beyond terrifying.

When he arrived at the airport, seven planes were waiting. The soldiers were shouting at everyone to get on a plane and Dad asked,

"Which one?"

"Anyone!" they shouted back. Another man asked where the flights would take us, and he got hit with the butt of a rifle for his curiosity. The flights were going to England, Sweden and Germany as well as Canada.

As the engines started, the captain announced the flight was going to England. A lot of Dad's friends were put on the other flights to other countries. Luckily his closest friends were on the plane with him.

Eventually, the plane landed in England and Dad was taken to Newbury where a camp had been erected to house the newly arrived Ugandan Asians. Dad volunteered to be the camp doctor and did such a good job that he was able to apply for a job in a GP surgery and got a job in Reading. He sent for us, and he and Mum bought a house and my brothers, and I moved in to start our lives in England.

Now, moving for the third time, Mum needed to make a new home for us all. Mum had trouble finding her feet when we arrived in the UK, so Dad went out to find out if there was anyone in the community who could help her settle in. Jay and Indira Kundalia were such a good help to Mum then visiting regularly and cooking with her. It really helped Mum to feel more at home. Dr Uncle Satish and Auntie Barfula were also an immense help to Mum, and we could walk to their house from ours. They were very kind and helped Mum get used to living in Reading. Auntie Sonu and Uncle Ranu were very close to us as well. We had met them at the local community centre for Asian people and they helped to assimilate us into the local community. Ramesh and Illa were also friends in those early days, and we are still the best of friends today. Mum quickly gained respect from the whole community due to her ability and skill in cooking delicious Gujarati food and for her permanent and captivating smile. She earned the nickname Kaki (Auntie). Everyone knew who you meant if you said Kaki. I am pretty sure that I got my project management skills from Mum. She was well respected and a brilliant organiser. People visited often and that made her enjoy living in Reading. She finally felt at home again after the terrible experience in Africa. After years of struggle and difficulties, Mum finally gained a great circle of friends to give her the joy in life back again. Now, she could relax and enjoy watching her boys grow up. She was happy and fulfilled once more and she even teased me about my long hair!

When I was a bit older, plans were made to visit Tanzania again and I was dead against that. I was old enough to be able to drag a chair to the work counter and climb up and get onto the top of the tall fridge. Mum asked me what I was doing and `I told her I did not want to go. She told me to get down and not be so silly. I knew that I would damage my leg if I jumped and I did, it I broke! I had to go to hospital and have my leg put in plaster of Paris. The family set off for Tanzania along with me who had a cast on!

A few months later, we returned, and Dad took us up Murchison Falls for a break. We drove there which took 5-6 hours. My oldest brother Ahmed took charge of me and comforted me. Dad found parking near the falls and got us all onto a boat trip all around the lake and the falls.

When we got back to the car, we started to head back to Kampala, a 6-hour drive and the journey was incredible. The sun was setting and the animals were gathering under the trees, out of sight. I said to Dad, "Where are all the animals?"

Just as I said that we came across a giraffe in the middle of the road. We also saw a gathering of vultures. We did not stop for anything to eat. Mum was a vegetarian and all that was on offer was chicken, of various types. so, we kept going!

I so admire all those people, like mum and dad who had to start all over again and I think that a lot of my resilience comes from what I experienced and how I saw them behave at that terrible time.

I was just old enough to start primary school when I arrived in the UK and Dad applied to the Southcote primary school, who accepted me. On the first day, I was so nervous, and I had reason to be because it was the first time I was to experience racism.

When I was eleven, I moved to senior school at Stoneham Secondary School. I played a lot of cricket, at school and I was good enough to be picked for the Berkshire 1st team. I used to open the batting with Gordon Greenwich. One of Dad's very closest friends, Nagin Kaka, had played for the Ugandan National Team but my Dad persuaded him to take up golf once they got to England. Nagin kaka had settled in London. Dad, as senior partner at his surgery, took every Wednesday afternoon off and demanded that Nagin Kaka join him on the golf course. Dad did not have to twist his arm as Nagin Kaka knew that Dad would cook for us all and the food was very good! We all looked forward to Wednesday afternoons. Sadly, we lost Nagin Kaka in 1989. It was this ritual on a Wednesday afternoon that introduced me to the love of cooking. I loved to watch Dad cook and always asked him to cook his lamb curry. I learned to cook seafood in a tasty and healthy way, and it has led to one of my passions in life - entertaining people. I love to set the table to a tee, just like The Ritz. I will talk to my guests about what they like to eat and find out the appropriate wine for the dish I am serving. I have now got 50 recipes for desserts I created when I was in the hospital for so long. Nowadays, I use less garlic and chilli and more herbs like parsley, mint and dill. People would call me up and ask me to marinate fish and meat for them to cook on their barbecue. My risotto is a wonder, and I love to cook that for people.

Chapter 2
Events Management

As further education loomed, I was determined to have enough money for University and to be able to go out at the weekends, so I got a Saturday job at a Jewish tailor's shop. I ended up selling lots of suits for him, mainly by changing the music he played in the shop. At that time men dressed smartly to go out. With a change of music to something a bit funkier I would help a chap pick a suit and I would say,

"That is a ten-to-two suit!"

"What do you mean?" he would say.

"That is the suit that you will be wearing when the last dance is playing at ten to two in the morning, and your thoughts turn to picking a lovely lady for that last dance."

"I see," the gentleman would say, "Well let me look in the mirror!"

"Never mind that, let me get you a lady who will tell you whether she would dance with you if you asked her in your ten to two suit." I would suggest.

That lady was Sophia. I had persuaded the tailor that we needed to employ an attractive lady saleswoman, who would flatter the customers.

Sophia was Italian - extremely attractive and elegant with a lovely personality. We started to go out for lunch periodically and we had such a laugh. We would compete to see who could sell the most suits. The prize would be 25-30% off something from the store. I was always a good-looking dude, but with a slick suit, I was unbeatable, even though I say it myself! You needed to be well dressed to get into a good nightclub. I made it my business to get to know the manager and the bouncers, so I never had to pay to go in.

Sanjay was someone I had known since I was 11. We went on holidays together and in the nightclub years, we would have competitions to see who got the loveliest girl in the nightclub. We were more like brothers. We did everything together; we went to the same bars and clubs. Our circle of friends got bigger and bigger. We went to all the top nightclubs in London. Sanjay now has three restaurant bars in Spain which he managed to set up in 6 months. I still phone him and give him tips on how to make good profit margins on certain dishes. I promised him that I would go and help him set up the restaurant and get suppliers. He lives with a lovely Spanish girl, and she has it all organised for him. I spoke to him recently and told him to look out for a great villa for me. I would consider retiring there. With Sanjay there, I would not be alone.

I was now at Reading College to study electronics. I made some life lifelong friends there and fortunately, six of us from the same year at college were subsequently admitted to Greenwich University. We still meet up!

The six of us loved entertaining and I was made the 'entertainment officer'. I would organise all sorts of events from dinner dances and boat parties to nightclub outings. I used to get them all to sell tickets and if they sold more than 50 tickets, they could attend free and could have five more tickets free, as well. They would recruit friends from other Universities and the events I put on soon got very well-known and tickets were sought after.

I hired a boat, Myuki from Japan, it was brand new, with a dance floor and DJ area. It would take 200-300 people. For the first dance night, I was sold out and when they wanted another boat party,

I phoned the boat owner and said,

"I know how much you made behind the bar for the last party, so don't think that you can charge me the same this time!"

He protested but I said,

"Look the next event is going to have a lot more affluent people attending. We're not talking bottle of beer and a glass of prosecco, we're talking bottles of your best champagne."

He saw it my way and I put away what I saved - 20%- into a separate account. After the function, I would pay him off. With the money I made, I took every friend out for dinner. The boys loved that and for the girls, I would lay on a shopping trip. I would hire a minibus to go to the East End. One girl told me she wanted a Chanel handbag, and I said,

"Sell 100 tickets and you will get one!"

She did it!

I remember that I had to take the boys to a men's outfitter because they looked so scruffy. They came out looking very slick.

"Lads, this is how you should always dress. This is the secret you always ask me about my success with women, looking good and treating them well." I said.

I bought lovely suede jackets for each of us, and we all wore them to the next function.

People used to say to me that I should have gone into Event Management and maybe in another life, I would have. I used to have carrier bags full of cash. I would put handfuls in my blazer, and I would hand over £200-300 to the barman and tell him to announce that the next drink was on me and all the girls could have a cocktail. I was popular and I even had a proposal from one of the girls I knew. I turned her down and now when I think back, it was the biggest mistake I made.

One of my close friend Ronnie from college, I still keep in touch with even after 20 years. He was regarded as a very intelligent young and today he is leading a very high executive role in one of the biggest banking firms. The time I spent with Ronnie at college, and he was admired and looked up by many because of his dedication to studies. He was a role model to many people, and I really wish if I could have made him my role model too. He was good looking Punjabi guy, and many girls desired to be with him for his personality and his calm attitude.

He always used to encourage me to study and attend lectures, and I helped him finding his next girlfriend.

Ronnie's words to Ajay:

Ajay was clearly the leader of our pack during college days and had an innate ability to create new friends and relationships across all facets of life – inside college, and out. A social animal at heart, he would forge relationships with so many people, it was a wonder how he had time to attend lectures and tutorials to achieve the grades he needed, to progress onto higher education, but he did so in style, charm and wit!

One of the times that I remember well was an event I organised at my first workplace at St Regis Paper Company. I made some great friends there and we still meet to this day. I took it upon myself to welcome new employees, and I was told to go along and see if I could do a deal for some entertainment for the staff of the business, with a local boat owner. I went to see him and said,

"I see that your boat is sitting there every night gathering mould. If it was on the move, it would not be so dirty!"

"We can pick a day that is convenient for you, and as it is in a residential area, we cannot be too late. What do you say?"

I told him where I worked and I managed to get a DJ, some fish and chips. I also arranged to have people picked up from work with the promise to bring them back to their cars again, at the end of the night.

The deal was done. The boat party finishing early suited me as we had a nightclub, Valbornes, that even had a hot tub, that we liked to go to! Champagne was cheap there and my friend Des Patel and I would often go there after the boat parties. We were quite naughty, really, but we had fun.

On the Move

I went to Spain in the year 2000 where I opened three businesses from scratch, in two years not speaking the language and getting to grips with tax and employment law to boot! I opened a restaurant, a supermarket and a takeaway selling Indian food. One of the chefs tried to hold me to ransom, thinking that I couldn't do without him. Turned out I could. Most of the customers preferred my food! But the building was unused during the day until I had a brain wave - by day it became a proper café for Brits with sandwiches, breakfasts, cakes and even homemade sausage rolls that were a huge hit. We had the best coffee machine on the coast, and we slowly got recognition. The local Spanish people began to love the idea of having their meals brought to them, too!

The supermarket was 300 ft sq. My lost leader was milk. The Brits hated UHT milk so to find fresh milk for them I went to a local farmer. That got people in there in droves and then I would hear the till ringing all day long as they snapped up other things that they missed from home which I sold

One of my friends from the UK gave me the idea of sourcing women's clothes from the UK taking advantage of end-of-season sales. I would fly into Manchester and fill a container with £2000 worth of end-of-season clothes - bras and knickers that were particularly requested. I told them that I would give them any size that they needed, and I told them that I was very good with cup sizes, not so much with mugs! It was a very lucrative sideline. I learned a lot about the type of clothing the expat ladies would like. I would pick up loads of light, colourful dresses and I would tease the ladies who bought them, saying that they should make sure the almost see-through material did not give them away! One of my employees said to me that I could sell sand to the Egyptians.

Chapter 3
Employment Journey

After I finished University, I struggled to find work until a temporary staffing agency finally got me an interview at the St Regis Paper Recycling Mill. Jim Lyle, the personnel manager at the time, saw me arrive in the car park and asked if he could help. We went up to Sue Lennon's office. She was sitting in a big leather armchair with a cigarette and G&T on the go. I put my hand out to shake hers and she said, "You must be Ajay." She asked me if I drank, and I said I did. She got her secretary to bring a special G&T for me (one with a bit more gin in it). She asked me if I wanted to smoke and told me not to be afraid to light up even though it was an interview. She offered me one of her More menthol cigarettes. I said I would loved one. Just then Valerie the secretary came in to find us both rocking in the armchairs drinks in hand and smokes on the go. She said, "It looks like Sue has found a new friend!"

Sue Lennon was my first boss at St Regis Paper Recycling Mill!!

I offered to show Sue what I had been studying at the University, but she waved my documents away saying, "Look, you are clearly a great personality, unflappable and you like Mores so you'll do for me. Can you start on Monday?"

I was to work in Accounts with Sylvia. On Monday morning, Sue introduced me to the staff. As I walked past Sylvia she said, "Hey Sue, who's this darkie?" When I laughed, she jumped up, hugged me, and said she did not mean it. I said, "Well you said it, so I think you meant it!" I was the start of a special relationship that often had us dissolving into uncontrollable laughter and getting up to more than our share of tricks.

'The darkie' became a standing joke that we played out. I remember when the new financial controller arrived.

He said,

"My name is Neil, I am the new financial controller."

"Pleased to meet you" Sylvia chirped, "Oh and meet the darkie, he is my assistant." Neil's face was a picture.

The company was on the river and included a lovely old house where the MD lived and where I eventually got an office. I would ring Sylvia from there and ask for a cup of tea. She would say "I'm not coming down to you snobs in the posh end, even though you are a darkie!"

My office was once the bedroom that the daughter of the house had slept in, overlooking the Koi carp pond. The MD would get me to count them, there were twelve in all.

Sue Lennon was a real party animal, and we always had lots of Christmas dos and barbeques. We would have a huge marquee up in the summer for our functions with tribute bands and all sorts of entertainment. Sue would always have Sylvia and me on her table as we always had the most laughs.

At one function, Sue whispered to me," Don't drink too much, The MD wants you to do a speech."

"Me? Why? That is usually the big boss's territory!" I protested.

"I know, Sue said, "But he has been watching you and thinks you would do a grand job." Sylvia and Sue were tickled that I was getting so nervous. Then the moment came, and I was introduced.

I took a big gulp of G&T and said, "Get me another drink Sylv, I'll need it."

"Who do you think I am, your goffer?" she said.

"No, but you are a whitie!" I quipped.

We always had our Christmas dos in a five-star hotel, and they would pay for the rooms for us to stay with our wives and girlfriends. On one occasion, I told Sue that I would see her at the bar at midday while our partners were in the rooms getting ready.

We would get trollied, but we would be down again by seven. Sue would change all the names at the table settings so that we three were sitting together. Everyone was invited and the whole company came.

When the do was over, I found myself at the bar with the IT director who had a high opinion of himself. His name was Robert Notley. At the do, if you had no money, anything you ordered could be put on the room bill, for the company to pay. Robert and I had a drink, and he put it on his room, telling the bartender it was room 411. I saw the opportunity for a great trick immediately. I told everyone to put everything they drank on room 411. I got Sylvia the best gin in the place, despite her protestations and put it on – you guessed it, room 411.

About three weeks later Sue asked me what room I had been in at the Christmas do, "Was it 411?"

"No I was in a first-floor room." I replied.

Sylvia was stifling a giggle and Sue said,

"You did something, didn't you?"

We told her what had happened and that it was Robert Notley's room. She said it was the best prank we had ever played.

Lots of other guys my age joined at the same time as I did, and we have stayed in touch ever since.

Phil Brown was my next boss when I came back from Spain. I was jobless and moneyless because of the recession. A friend of mine, Steve Hawks, called and said he had a project, and he could take me on as a contractor, so I joined Causeway with Phil Brown as the CEO at the time. I have to say that I learned a lot from watching Phil, in those days at Causeway. He had a knack of dealing with the most awkward of customers and really educated me in how to manage customer expectations. He told me that I could come on board to help to get one of their clients, SSE under control. From that time, we had each other's back, always. Steve Hawks now lives in Singapore with his lovely wife and two daughters. We have such a bond that he flew back to see me when I had my stroke.

On that day, however, I met the current project manager, Jeff Hobden. I told him that I was not trying to take his job. As we got acquainted, the manager of SSE called, yelling at Jeff as she had become accustomed to doing. Her name was Andrea Marriott

I took the phone from Jeff and told her I was on the project now and that I would be conducting all meetings at 4 pm and added that she should not be late. I also said we needed to impose a 3-month deadline to have the project completed. I did it successfully and Phil Brown was ecstatic that the project was completed and he could start making some money from a customer who had initially refused to pay, due to the inability of previous project managers to complete the projects. The MD of SSE asked me up to Glasgow to go over the way I had handled the project.

The flight was at 6 am. We flew to Glasgow and rented a car, and Jeff Hobden drove. We got to the head office and the receptionist knew we were coming. We went into the MD's office. He was rocking in the chair with his feet on the desk, just as I had once seen Sue Lennon do.

The MD complimented me for about 15 minutes about how I had approached and completed the project.

"Ajay took this project by the scruff of the neck and got it done." Phil Brown said.

The MD took the contract and signed it.

"So now we can have some lunch," Phil said.

"I haven't arranged lunch for you." The MD said.

We went to the canteen, and Phil was not impressed. We had a sandwich. He said to me. "In the future, Ajay, you are going to lead the projects, and while you're at it, make sure there is a decent lunch available!"

Phil was pleased that the contract had been signed, plus we now had a clause that would raise the amount paid, with inflation. I ended up delivering thirty-five projects for SSE and Causeway. Then came contracts with Balfour Beatty and other big hitters. It was an exciting time and a time that finely honed my organisational skills.

Carol worked with me at Causeway as an account manager. She and Ray Massay (her husband) have been good friends of mine for a long time and were very supportive when I had my stroke. And Carol was kind enough to write a reference for my book. I learned a lot about business from Carol and more than that, through the years, we have become close friends. She is more like a sister to me now. She has made me an extremely proud brother by achieving a high level in her sector of employment career and becoming a doctor. Now she is inspiring a lot of other women to come and work in a male oriented industry of construction.

Carol's personal Tribute to Ajay:

"Working in a sector where all the faces are male, and white was very daunting for me 30-plus years ago and the challenges are still here today. I remember working for a busy construction tech company in the early 2000s, driving around the UK and showing some of the top 100 contractors the reasons why technology was going to improve the bottom line. It was 2010 when. as part of another restructure, I was introduced to Ajay. "Great project management expertise and good with customers" the head of Professional Services said. Following several strategic acquisitions, we needed someone to help the customer remain focused and to give our teams the time to implement change.

Ajay and I clicked straightaway, well with him being someone of colour, I didn't feel alone anymore. We worked together on some of the biggest accounts having challenging conversations and aggressive timescales. We dealt with many personalities that helped us deliver success.

We also had fun, Ajay loves to keep the team upbeat, from sharing his mouth-watering recipes from the weekend to the jokes he shared.

I remember a time when we had a high-powered meeting with one of our biggest clients. Our CEO was going to be joining us, so we knew the pressure was on. We met at a coffee shop 2 hours before the meeting to ensure we had all our notes aligned. In those days, we were working on many projects around the country so getting together sometimes was often last-minute-dot com. I was very nervous, not about the meeting but because the boss was going to be there. Ajay could see this and kept saying, "Relax we've got this". He was so right but sometimes you just need that friendly voice and someone who's not talking BS.

With the team, Ajay and I had some great times, lunches and evening meet-ups too. Very generous with sharing we were able to use his Spanish apartment at "mates rates" which was such a lovely experience.

Life has changed from those days, but despite where we are now and what Ajay has gone through, he's shown so much strength as he works through everything he has had to face and I am so inspired by where he is today. I am proud to have him as my dear friend and brother. The future is his, and I do not doubt that although it may be on a different path, the path that has been gifted to him, he will make the most of the change of direction and I know that he will be the champion he is and get on with life."

Avtar Baines

I took Avtar on and he started on a Monday. He came to my office, but he looked awful. I asked what was wrong. He replied, "the only place I could find to stay was a bed and breakfast. I said, "You look very tired."

He replied, "I haven't slept all day and night."

Because it was his first day, we had a lot to catch up on, and I asked him to walk me home that night. He asked, "Why do I need to drop you off at home when you have a car?"

I said, "Don't ask questions, just walk me home."

I found five minutes to phone my wife to tell her to get the small room ready as Avtar was going to stay with us.

I asked Avtar to pack his bags and asked if the landlady of the B n B was fully paid for.

"Yes, all paid up. Why do you want me to pack my bags? Where are we going?"

I replied "You are moving in with me until further notice!"

At that time, I had two kids and a five-bedroom house.

Avtar asked if everybody would be okay with him moving in.

I replied, "Everything is okay; you don't have to worry about all this. You will be very welcome."

Eventually, we got home, and the moment we opened the door, I saw my two kids (Krishan and Kinari) running towards the door. Krishan shouted "Daddy, daddy, is that your friend's car?" Krishan is as fond of cars as Avtar is!

Avtar asked Krishan "Hey, young man, do you like sports cars?"

Krishan nodded with the biggest grin on his face.

Avatar said, "Krishan, if you finish your homework and meal on time, then I will take you for a ride in my car, for sure!"

From then on, Avtar and I became very good friends. We worked together, we partied together, ate together and as the months passed, we realised we had so many things in common that he became like family.

During the time he stayed with us, we had our third child named Nishal. Avtar used to take care of him for us sometimes, feeding him, changing his clothes, and bathing him and they became close. That's how we made the journey from strangers to brothers, for which I will always be grateful.

Chapter 4

Family Life

My mum never recovered from the death of one of my brothers and she was very keen on me getting married. When I told her that I was seeing a girl from the University she insisted that I make some kind of declaration to save her and her family from disgrace. I did that because that is our custom.

I married that lady, who is now my ex. From the beginning, it became clear that she was after whatever money she could get, and it was also noticeable that she had no respect for my mother, whom she used to swear at. My mother was ecstatic when we had our first child - her first grandson. She would come around at weekends to try and help only to be told to f-off. I always respected my ex's family and helped them financially and in any other way I could. I told her I expected the same respect for my family, from her. The response I got was hurtful. She told me that my mother had her nose in our business. She said she did not know why she came to our house on the weekend. I told her that Mum came to help her, to clean and cook. Also, Mum loved my son so much, they had such special times together. My ex was happy about that because with her baby taken care of, she was free to go out. I do remember one Saturday morning, my mum asked what she should cook for our evening meal. My ex snapped back that she was going to a restaurant with some colleagues at 6 pm. Mum told her she would still be cooking, and that dinner would be at 8 pm. It took my ex

1.5 hours to get ready and then she came down demanding that all the windows and doors be opened so she would not smell of curry.

She said she would be back at 8 pm but then turned up at midnight. My mum called out when she heard the stairs creak, asking my ex if it was her. My ex flew into a rage, asking her what it had to do with her what time she came in? Mum asked my ex why she had not called to say she would be late as we had been waiting to eat with her.

I came from where I was sleeping to see what the commotion was. I told my ex she was out of order. Mum was clearly just worried that something might have happened to her because she was so late.

My ex told me to take my mother home on Sunday.

"OK, I'll do that. Why should she stay here to be insulted by you? But there is one thing I need you to do," I said.

"What?" she snapped.

"I need you to be out of the house when I come back from dropping mum, I need a break, a 'half term' Go back to your parents and leave my son with me for my mum and me to look after."

But when I came back, she refused to go.

"Look I need a break!" I shouted," you stay out till all hours and then you're abusive and rude when Mum speaks to you. I have had enough!" That was 1995.

At that time, I was working for St Regis still. As a work force, we worked and played hard. We started Christmas from the beginning of December. My ex hated me being picked up and taken to do's. I worked hard and I was ambitious. I wanted the IT manager job. My ex messed me up so badly I could not concentrate. I lost that promotion.

One day I realised that if there was going to be any hope of saving our relationship we needed to get away for a few days. I suggested we go to our place in Murcia, a property on the golf course in Spain.

"Just you and me?" she said.

"Just you and me." I nodded

I worked out a surprise trip for her and took her to Rome and Murcia, Amsterdam and finally to Thailand. It was a belated honeymoon for five-weeks. We travelled from north to south and all the islands in Thailand. I paid for everything because I did not want her to say she took me, and I booked with Kuoni. They liked my itinerary so much that they asked if they could use it as a honeymoon package in their brochure.

I arranged all sorts of special trips like a visit to an elephant sanctuary in Chang Mai and a trip down the river with an experience of feeding the elephants, too. We went on to Ko Samui.

A local guy in Chang Mai had told me that if we went to Ko Samui, we should hire one of the little scooters and then find a waterfall in the middle of the island where we could jump off the top. We did as he said and having found a tour guide, we climbed up the side of the waterfall. I noticed the trees I passed had tropical fruit. Our tour guide picked some papaya for us and said once we finished the last piece we would jump. I could not eat it quick enough and my ex was nervous. I said,

"Let me go first and if you hear me screaming you will know if it is safe or not!" The guide gave me a signal, and I ran off the top holding my knees up to my chest. It was so exhilarating. I swam to where the water was falling - it was such a special and invigorating experience. My ex, however, was having none of this.

"I didn't come here for this; I want to go to the beach." She moaned.

The tour guide, however, took it in his stride and said,

"Come on, we will go to the beach for a BBQ." My ex sulked the whole way, complaining that she did not know what the BBQ would be like.

We arrived to find a whole barracuda was cooking on the BBQ, the length of it across the coals. The tour guide's mother cut it into steaks.

"I just wanted to go to the beach." My ex pouted.

"For God's sake!" I said, "Have a look at where you are, the sand is beneath your feet - you're at the beach!" We had sweet potato and roasted coconut next, and I felt so full, but my ex was still not happy. After picking at her food, she said,

"I want to go somewhere to eat. I'm still hungry!"

"Come on!" I said, "Let's help tidy up. Then we can go for a swim."

We had our swim but when we came out, the tour guide's mother called us over. She had cooked a local speciality, first grating coconut, then draining the milk to make the most amazing gooey coconut chunks - quite like an Indian sweet dish. I told her it was fantastic.

She told me that everything was natural. My ex said,

"It's Ok, nothing spectacular."

I was mortified and so I hugged the lady, calling her Aunty and I told her that she had treated us so well and her son had been wonderful too; she truly was a treasured Aunty.

She was crying with joy. She held my hand, and she said,

"You are a good man, please, before you go, teach my son a few things."

"He doesn't need to be taught anything!" I said.

I said to my ex "Pass me my wallet." I took out about £20-30 that but Aunty flatly refused to take it. Eventually, I slipped it into her apron pocket. It would mean so much, I knew that. My ex was appalled at what I had done.

I still wanted to help clean up for Aunty, and I was doing that, although the guide said we should leave it. I asked what they would do with the remains of the barracuda.

I told him he should call the family down to finish it up.

"No, mum wants you to take it!" He protested. But I would not be persuaded. I reminded him that our resort was full board so we would have no opportunity to eat the fish. It was so delicious that I could not bear to see it wasted and the thought of his young nephews, nieces and cousins enjoying such a feast would make me so happy.

This was, in fact, the sort of thing that was typical of me, I always want to help and do my bit, but my ex hated that, or any generosity I showed anyone. I never could understand that.

Our young guide rowed us back to the resort and as we got close to the shore, I decided I would jump in before we reached land. My guide said I should be careful, but I felt no fear. I could see a rock below me in the crystal-clear water and thought I would put my foot on it just to get my balance. Unfortunately, my 'rock' turned out to be a sea urchin! It was pure agony as its spines plunged into my foot. I screamed and my guide did not hesitate, he jumped in and got me over to a rock as he rowed to shore to find lemons, that are supposed to ease the pain. It took him ten minutes to take out all the spines. My ex? Well, she sat unmoved and unresponsive, on the boat. She paid me no attention at all.

Once he got me back to the resort, despite the agony, I was determined to me pay him for the day.

"You have already given money to my Mum." He protested but I made him take the money. I really appreciated his kindness and the way he had gone the extra mile for us. It had been a magical experience, having the barbeque and I knew that it was something that not many people would get to experience. The disapproval from my ex was almost palpable.

The manager of the hotel told us that if the guide had not acted quickly when I had stepped on the sea urchin, I would have been in serious trouble.

My ex was furious that I had given the young man the money and that was typical of her. Even a fabulous trip to Florida that I arranged once, barely raised a smile from her. I had intended to buy a holiday home with a swimming pool when we got there but trouble started even before we left the airport. As we sat in the terminal before we left for Florida, she said she was going to buy some chewing gum from Boots. She actually went for a pregnancy test. She did the test and came back to announce that she was pregnant with our third child. I was astonished but delighted too.

On board the stewardess who was looking after us in first class asked if we would like a drink. I told her that we were celebrating as I had just discovered that we were expecting another baby. She was delighted for us and asked what she could get for my ex, who said that she wanted a Tia Maria. Unfortunately, there was none on board. My ex was furious. She said angrily,

"What kind of first class is this if you don't have any Tia Maria?"

I knew then that we were starting to drift apart, I could not take her attitude, her ingratitude.

The day we came back from Thailand was the day Princess Diana died. I had switched on the TV and was trying to follow what had happened. But my ex was not having that. She told me to sort out the luggage.

One thing we agreed on was that we would get the best flowers for Princess Di and we did. She arranged to take the flowers to London going along with some of her friends. She said she would be back by 8.30 in the evening. I told her I could cope while she was away and asked her to keep in touch, especially if she was going to be late. She did not keep in touch and arrived back at midnight.

The first thing she said to me "Have you done the washing?" I said I had done that and fed the children and put them to bed but had eaten nothing, myself. In the thirteen years of marriage, she never made me so much as one cup of tea in the morning. Meanwhile I would get ready for my day every morning, wanting to look smart and make the best impression. Work was about a one-and-a-half-hour drive away.

I suppose, typical for a man, I did not say anything to anyone else. Maybe if I had, they could have helped. She left me in February, 2018. I never heard from her again. I heard plenty about her, however. She went on the local radio station, completely assassinating my character and discrediting me and people told me that she had been on Facebook doing the same. She has also posted a photo of herself, scantily dressed, with the caption, 'Come on boys, if you want it, come and get it!' Quite something for someone in our culture! She was really scraping the bottom of the barrel by that time.

She also posted a picture of me on Facebook, defaced it and wrote over it," You f****g prick". She then went ahead and tagged everyone so that not only me, but all my friends saw it. People would contact me and tell me what she was up to. It was embarrassing and sad to see someone stoop so low.

There were good times, of course, especially with the children because my children have always been a great joy to me. Growing up, Nishal was a comedian and looked after his sister so well. He adored her and would do anything for her. I do hope that closeness endures. My son Krishan was a great swimmer and he and I would go deep-sea diving together. We loved to go deep. One year, Kinnari, my daughter, bought us an underwater camera. She took some photos of me and Krishan swimming underwater. I wanted to ensure that they were not scared of water. They could all swim, although their mother would not get in the water. Luckily, they were all comfortable swimming and loved the water.

Kinnari is the light of my life. She is such a beautiful girl and at the moment she is living in London with her university friends. She studied Biology and started the course just when I had my stroke. I was very impressed with how stoic she was during my illness. She got on with her studies, weathered COVID and came out with a first in Biology. Kinnari has always loved kids and took a job in a nursery, initially helping out the chef. She did so well that the parents warned the bosses not to lose her. She has such a good reputation for her kindness and integrity. She manages her money so well and I encourage her to see as much of London as she can, while she is there. She walks everywhere and will often find an out-of-the-way restaurant and get me to come up for a meal. I will be doing the same property deal for my daughter as I am doing for her brothers.

Kinnari loved snorkelling. I would tell her to hold her breath and down we would go, and I would point out all the fish to her. She was very sporty and when we came back from Spain, she joined a football team. Her coach, Simon O'Leary and I would talk for hours in the pub about football. He took the team from the bottom of the division to winning the cup, two years running. Kinnari won several awards.

My eldest son Krishan is 27 and really stepped up after my stroke and was my full-time caregiver for the first year. He is a car salesman for Toyota and has become their top salesman. He had a target to sell 70 cars in a month and would sell that number in a fortnight! He has excelled in his career and I am very proud of him. I have told him that when I am back on my feet, we will get him a flat that he can live in or rent out.

My second son, Nishal is now 24. He was working for Amazon in a distribution hub and is now looking for an office job. He did very well at Talk Talk and picked everything up very quickly so I am sure he will do well. He has always helped me out when I was moving, for instance. He would take me shopping. He's very practical. Nishal manages his money well and we are working on how to get him a good investment home. We will make it work. It would be the same thing as with Krishan, a flat that they could make money from.

Unfortunately, my ex was not on the same page as regards future-proofing our children's lives. She does not really give them any useful advice and worse she pours scorn on anything that I say. I have my children in my will, everything is divided equally. They make me very proud.

---⊷⊷◄◊►⊷⊷---

Chapter 5

Resilience After My Stroke

On the 28th of March 2019, my birthday, I had a stroke. I had gone to work and had a meeting with Phil Brown.

He said, "I hear it is your birthday. Are you taking us for a drink?"

"Why not, I said!" Someone was leaving that day, so it was to be a dual event.

As we enjoyed our first round, my colleagues started asking me if I was OK. I was slurring and they had never heard me do that before, not after one glass of wine. I was asking for water. Then Ian Shelton noticed my face had dropped and asked for a comfortable chair. Another colleague, Jon sat me down and called an ambulance and said that he thought I was having a stroke. The ambulance crew confirmed that when they arrived. I was taken to Royal Berkshire Hospital and a CT scan identified a clot in the middle of my brain. A good friend of the family Dr Ramesh Naik came to my aid and organised for me to be moved to John Radcliff Hospital in Oxford for an emergency operation, where they took out the right side of my brain. The operation started at 9 pm and finished at midday the next day. My brothers were there the whole time. They were faced with the awful choice of me having an operation that might cause some disability or not having the procedure, which would come with even more risk of disability. I could not speak for myself. Thank goodness they chose the operation. I found all this out a long time after I came out of the hospital.

Much later, I learnt of all that could have happened to me as a result of the stroke. Any part of my body from head to toe, could have developed problems and lost function. I could have been paralysed for the rest of my life or even lost the capacity to speak. Thank God for the timely intervention and care,

The process of recovery was as strenuous as the weeks in the hospital. Frustrating with difficulties all along the way. Some of the most important factors that help in this process are the emotional ones like one's own motivation and ability to stick to the therapy sessions. Next comes the early start to a rehabilitation program and the skill of the rehabilitation team. And most importantly, social factors like the support of friends and family.

Fortunately for me, I had learnt the courage and resilience to recover from my early years and the team of therapists who so cheerfully nursed me back to health was as good as they come.

Ever since, I have always been full of gratitude to everyone involved with what happened that awful day. I was in John Radcliffe for 12 weeks and then Caversham Ward for rehabilitation for another 12 weeks. The medication was almost worse than the stroke, it gave me very bad dreams that I could have sworn were real. In one dream I dreamt that a Russian guy had shot me in the leg. I called the nurse over to see the blood, I was so convinced. The consultants realised that I was being affected by the medication that was making me dredge up memories of other times. Then there was a dream about my eldest son and my daughter. It was a very hot day, and they were visiting. I asked if they had been to Vietnam and I told them to look out of the window to see another hospital and football stadium that I said they could go to, later

I was eventually taken off those medicines and they put me on antidepressants. The stress of what my ex had done on top of everything else meant that I had to be locked in at times, as I just wanted to end it all. I shared this with the psychotherapist, and she talked me out of it all. I reassured them that I was OK, and that with my daughter doing her degree, I would not put her through another trauma of her father's suicide. I always tell people I am not afraid of dying and that is true.

I actually died twice in that year., When I had my stroke, I could not work and could not pay the mortgage in Spain. My ex was liable to pay half. Asit, my brother was a huge help at that time Asit contacted my bank manager, who said that I had 125,000 euros outstanding, half of which was the responsibility of my ex-wife. The manager asked for all my medical documents and then went to Spain to plead my case with the bank there, who said that they would wipe the mortgage and repossess the flat. It was a huge weight off my shoulders. They could do no more than that. The manager there told my brother that the backlog of payments (some 6 months) would have to be cleared and then the repossession could take place. It took so much effort from my brother with phone calls and faxes, emails and endless tasks. The result was that I could never buy in Spain again - and my ex? Well, she got off scot-free and not a word of thanks for the work that my brother did to get the best possible result for us. My ex cut me off once I had the stroke showing her true colours once again.

I had to keep going, I had to use all my resilience to keep me moving forward one painful step at a time, supported by my brothers and completely abandoned by my ex-wife.

Several people deserve my special thanks. Of course, my son, Krishan who cared for me so well in the first year after my stroke. Then there is Amit, my oldest brother who, since the day of my operation has encouraged me to get better and managed my paperwork and all the doctors. Equally my sister-in-law Romma, Amit's wife has been a tower of strength. She would bring me some Indian food in the evenings, warmed up as she knew that I did not enjoy the hospital food at all. I can truly say that without them I would not be here now. I feel often that there is nothing I could ever do to make up even a fraction of what they have done for me. I will always be eternally grateful.

Naveed and Negs, his wife, who met at nursery school and went to the same schools all the way along and then college were friends of mine and Naveed would come and sit with me in his lunch break for an hour. He did that virtually every other day. He would never wake me up but often, I would wake and find him there. We would talk about college days and when Negs came along with him, she would say that when I was better, I must visit them.

Beej Patel, my golfing buddy, phoned and checked up on me and if I was feeling low, he would take me out to dinner. He would get me out talking to friends because he knew that would always brighten me up.

Simon O'Leary was the coach of my daughter's football team. He loved Indian food and would bring food that he had cooked to me and would sit and chat for hours.

Then there was Setal Kundala and all her children. Setal took me on a holiday of a lifetime during my rehab. She rented a beautiful cottage with decking, in Devon. The sun shone and it was lovely. She massaged my hand so much that for the first time in years, I could open my fingers and catch a ball and throw it back again. I had known her since our youth, when we would go out together at night. I would take care of her and get her into nightclubs without paying. She was just like a sister to me. Her five children also brought me great joy during that time.

Dave Morris is a college friend who came to the hospital every day to take me for a walk and if it was cold, he would bring his big thick coat for me to wear. We are still very close, and his wife Joe invites me for exceptional dinner which she cooks.

Rodney Chandler and I studied together for over 30 years, and we both had a great passion for music and dancing. Jim Peacock was another one of the gangs, and our DJ. Andy Anguson who was also at university and used to help Jim set everything up and became a DJ himself in the end. Wayne Smith (Minter) was another school friend who never came to woodwork classes, but now, bizarrely, he is one of the best wood carvers I have known! He made me a walking stick and remains a really good friend.

Alay was part of my extended family, but I always thought of him as a very close friend. He would phone and check up on me and we had wonderful weekend holidays together as we had very similar interests.

Ramesh Naik, my consultant surgeon, is still in touch and I call him uncle. Without his knowledge and experience, I would not have had the operation that saved my life. Ila, his wife cooks the best banana loaf. She used to bring it to me in the hospital, and I still tease her about that now. My eyes would light up when she bought in another delicious home baked cake.

Emma Peppiatt was a stunning work colleague, and she visited me in the hospital on numerous occasions giving me lots of positivity that kept me going. When I was working, I would go in early just to spend time with her. She was as charming as she was beautiful. Her support after my stroke was something I was so grateful for. Her arrival in the ward was always like a breath of fresh air, a bright light in the gloom!

Aaron Ferdinand was another work colleague. We had worked together on various accounts, with some of the most awkward customers. He would always take me along because he knew that I wouldn't take any nonsense. I would take control of the situation and let them know in no uncertain terms that we would not be messed around. We spent many evenings in London together. Aaron loved to give people nicknames and he was the one who nicknamed me 'Magnet.' He gave me that nickname because he thought I was a true magnet to ladies. He once called me that in a meeting and from that day onwards, my CEO always called me by my nickname too. In return, I called Aaron MM (Master Magnet.). While I was in hospital, he kept in touch with me to check if there was anything I needed. He has been a true friend.

Another friend, Ian Shelton, who was with me when I had my stroke and who was a tower of strength after it, wrote the following:

"It was very shocking and distressing to see Ajay on the night he had his stroke, and on subsequent hospital visits. Ajay was always the life of the party, so to see him with lots of tubes attached and often sedated, was incredibly difficult.

What has happened since has been remarkable. It would have been very easy to give up and accept the life that fate had dealt him, but Ajay was never going to do that. Through hard work and determination, I could see both his physical condition and his mental awareness gradually improve over time. He has good days and bad days, but Ajay has learnt to cope with using just one hand for day-to-day tasks, and his brain (and wit!) are as sharp as ever. He works at this constantly and the results speak for themselves. He is an inspiration."

Ian Shelton

Chapter 6

At a Crossroads – Decision time

I developed a deeper passion for music while I was in the hospital, and I play my music on my Alexa every day. Part of my brain training is to get Alexa to refuse to play any music unless I can tell her the title and the artist. I love to meditate, too. Nowadays, I find I have drawn on my project management skills to keep me going. After my stroke, I would sit at home doing nothing and I decided that would not do. I decided to write several books and set myself goals. The first book was called Perseverance the second book Resilience and the third book, which I am working on now, is my autobiography.

I promised myself to make someone happy every day, make someone smile and to make someone laugh as well. So far, I have succeeded! My nurse is often doubled up with laughing so hard. I do forget things a bit, but I use association to remember. For instance, my nurse is called Bonnie, and I decided she would be Bonnie, and I would be Clyde!

The main reason I wanted to write the books was to inspire and encourage people who'd had strokes. I encourage baby steps and to keep going, little by little. I want to give people hope and a chance to see that you can get there.

The books were the challenge for this year and next year, my challenge will be to drive again. I will have to take another test. There is help for people like me and modifications that can be made to the car. I also want a companion, but I am housebound so that will be a challenge.

I always tell people that talking can be the best medicine. Talking to old friends about the good old days makes me happy. With a car, I will be able to visit them. Some of them came to visit every day during their lunch break and I miss seeing them! It would be great to get in a car and go and catch up with them again. We always have such fun together. daily.

After my stroke, I knew that I had to look at how I could change the way I lived and make serious lifestyle changes: I gave up red meat and now eat white meat and fish. I walk a lot more and I stopped drinking eleven months ago. I use a lot of meditation, brain games, puzzles and quizzes I was prepared to give up things I loved doing. I have missed all my friends' 50th birthday parties. I have not been out at night to wine bars or clubs either. All this is because I know I was given a second chance, and I want to make the most of that.

I realised as well how important it was to be in touch with friends and family. Catching up has been like medicine to me and I really enjoy talking about old times. I love a reunion, too, whether it be school, university or golf. We do not walk alone on this planet, my friends and family are as important to me as the air I breathe and I will never forget the contribution they have all, in their own way, made to my life. Very sadly, we lost my ex-father-in-law on Christmas day, 2024. I was so fond of him, and I remember the many times we used to cook together. I would have visited him in the hospital had I known he had been taken ill, but perhaps the proudest moment was when a friend of the family put on Facebook that my children had really rolled their sleeves up to help during the period of mourning.

I have recently met someone online who is of the same caste as me and who lives in Florida. She is keen for me to visit. Fortunately for my ex she was also in the right caste category and so she had my mum's backing. There is also a story that my dad actually delivered my ex, by some chance, in Uganda. I am not sure how true it is though.

I was always very good at rustling up a meal. I had to be, as my ex was never interested. I cooked for the kids a lot and I loved it. My talent was taking whatever we had and conjuring up a lovely meal from even the most meagre supplies. I am very much looking forward to writing my recipe book. I have some very interesting recipes to share!

After my stroke, life came to a sudden pause. I went from being constantly on the go in a busy job to just sitting at home, doing nothing — it was a complete shift, and honestly, quite tough to adjust to.

But slowly, things started to change — thanks to the unwavering support from **Autumn Care**. With their help, I began to feel like myself again. They encouraged me to take small steps forward and showed me that recovery could also be a journey of rediscovery. That gentle push helped me see I could start making better use of my time.

I'd always been curious about **AI** (Artificial Intelligence), but I never really understood how it worked. So, I decided to dive in — I spent two months learning through Google, navigating things on my own, and eventually completed a basic course. That small success was such a confidence boost. It reminded me that I was still capable of learning, growing, and doing more.

That confidence led me to explore further, and now I'm learning about solar farming — something I hope can help others, especially those in need, while contributing to a more sustainable future.

Honestly, I owe this new sense of purpose to Autumn Care. Their dedication not only helped me heal physically but also emotionally. They taught me how to manage everyday tasks with one hand — but more importantly, they helped me believe that my life wasn't over; it was just taking a new direction. And every day, that belief keeps me going, reaching for more.

EARLY YEARS

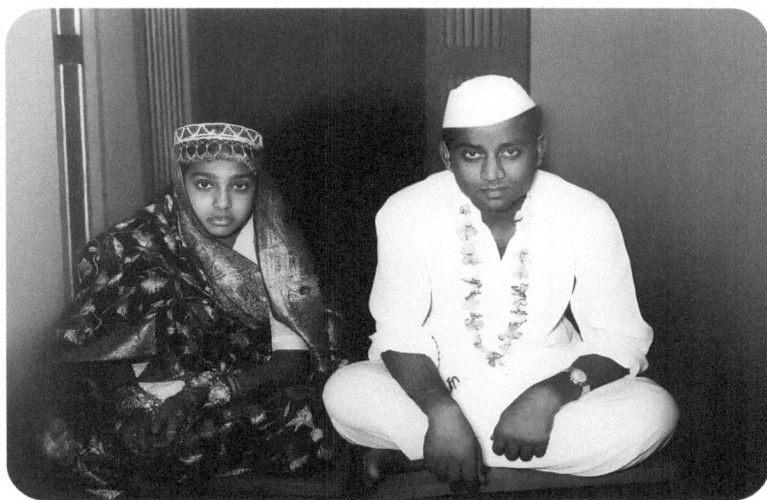

Mum and Dad's Marriage Picture

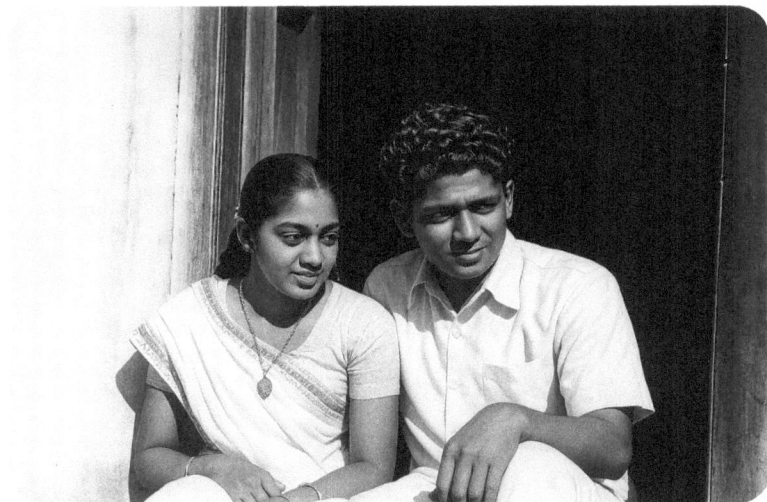

Mum and Dad enjoying their first house in Gulu, Uganda

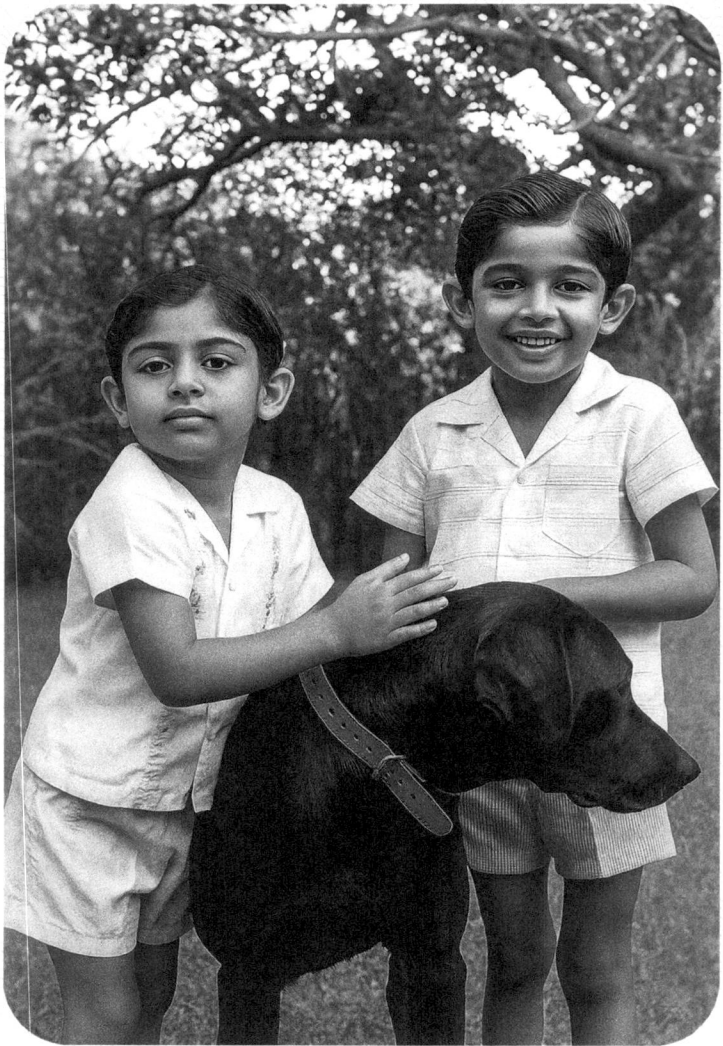

Me and Akhil Bhai with our first pet dog

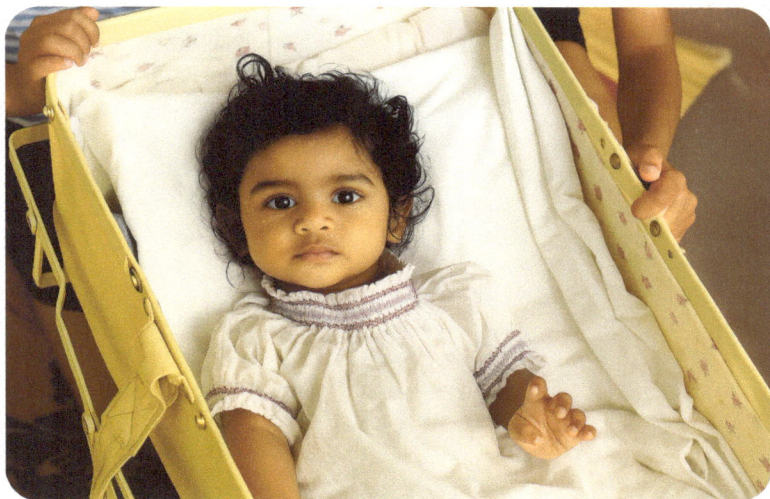

Cutest baby in all of Kampala

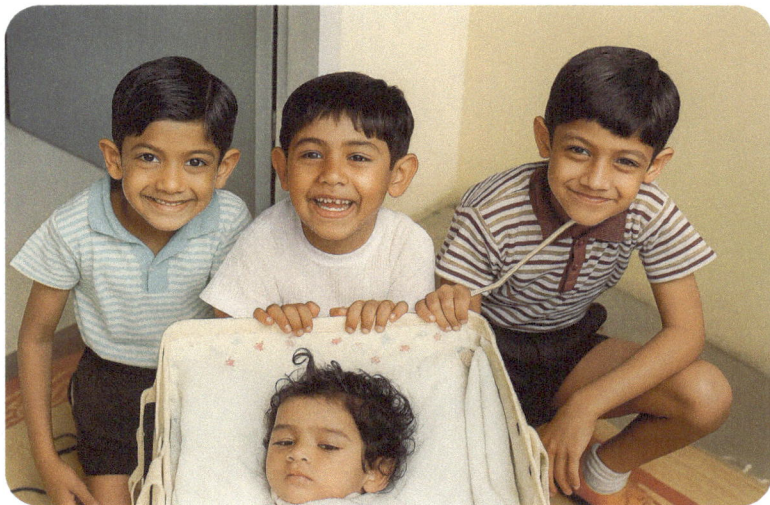

4 Brothers

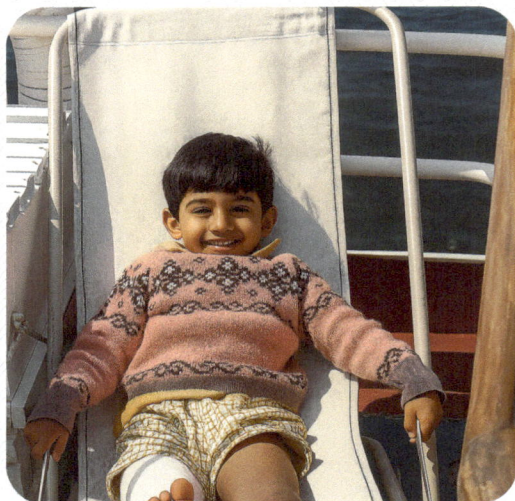

Me relaxing with the broken leg

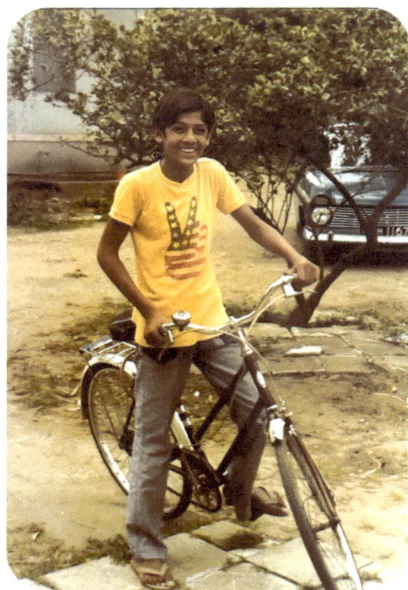

Amit Bhai enjoying his cycling lessons

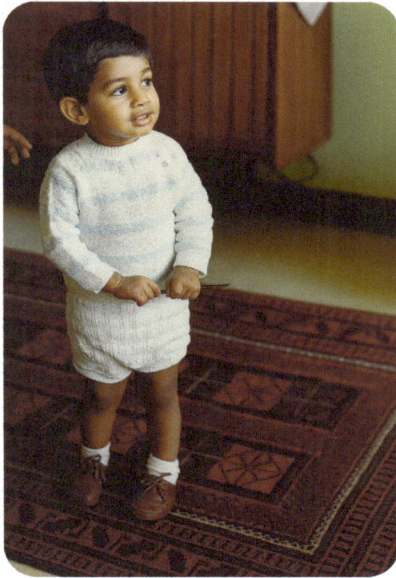

On my way to kitchen with a knife in hand

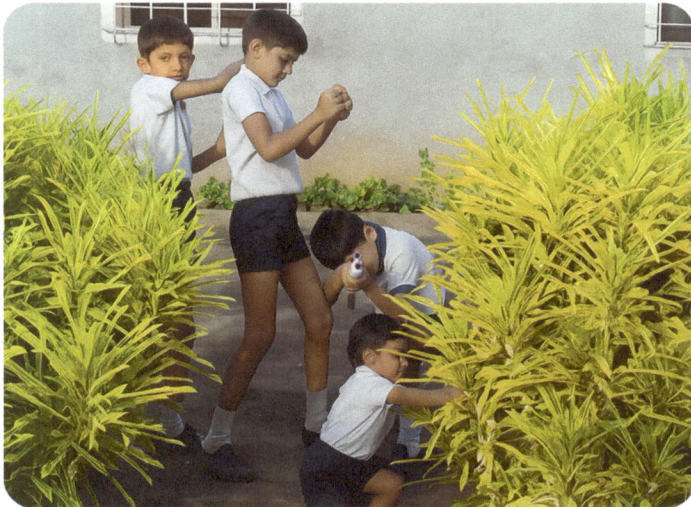

We playing our usual outdoor games

WHAT HEALING
LOOKS LIKE

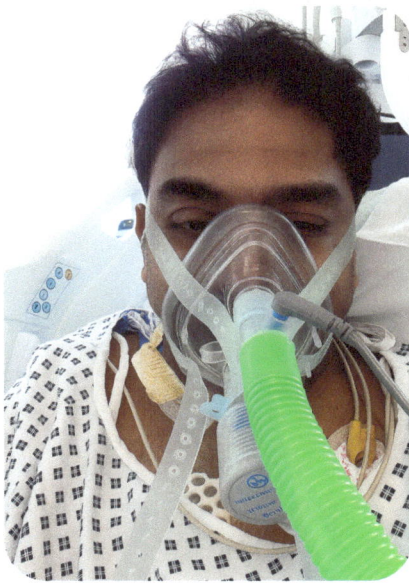

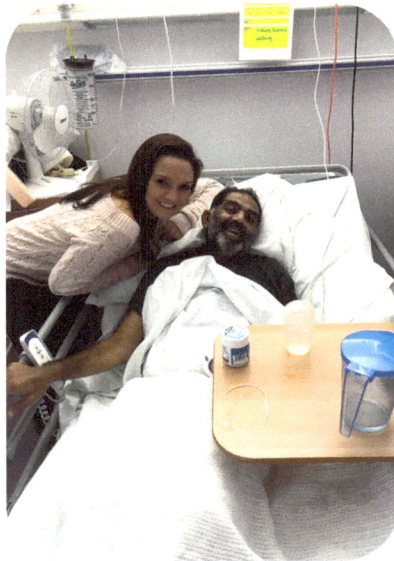

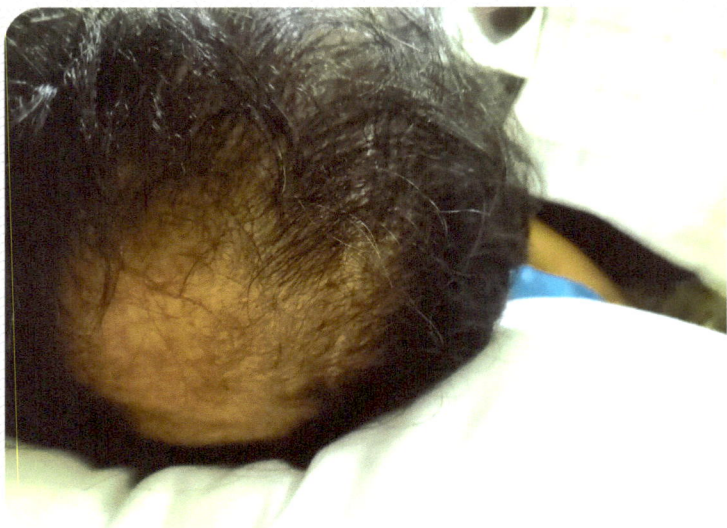

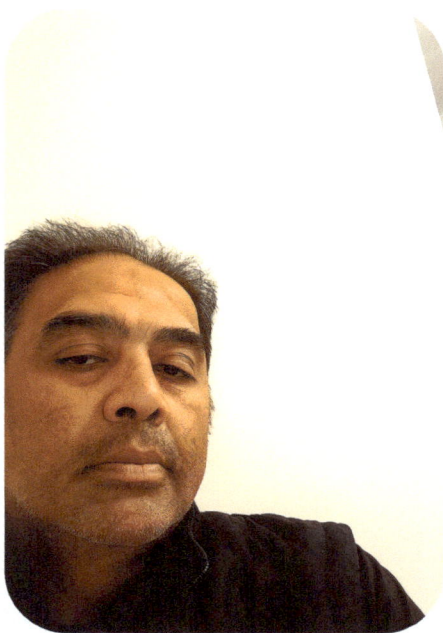

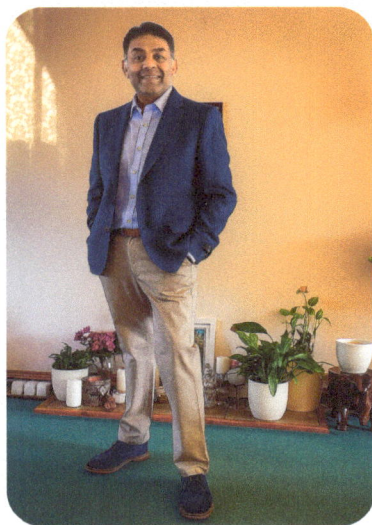

Me as usual looking the part when going out socialising

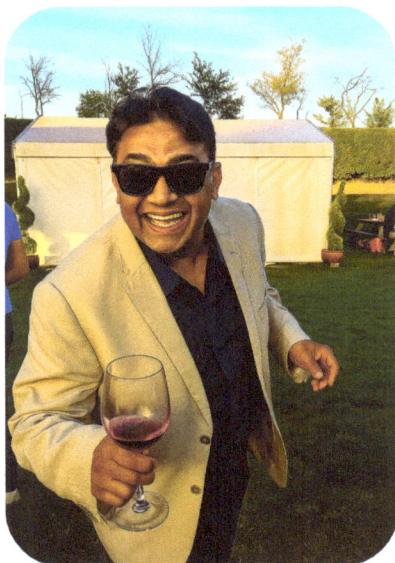

Me showing off my usual personality

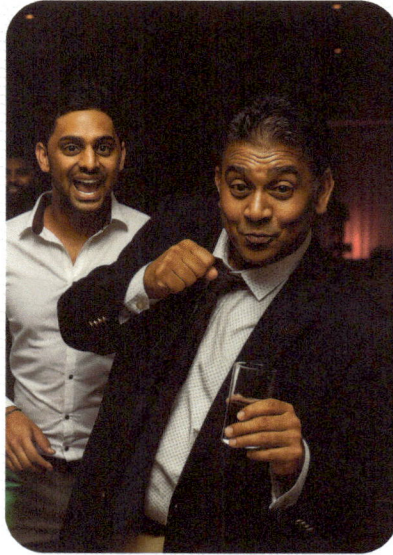

Me auditioning for Mr Bond 007

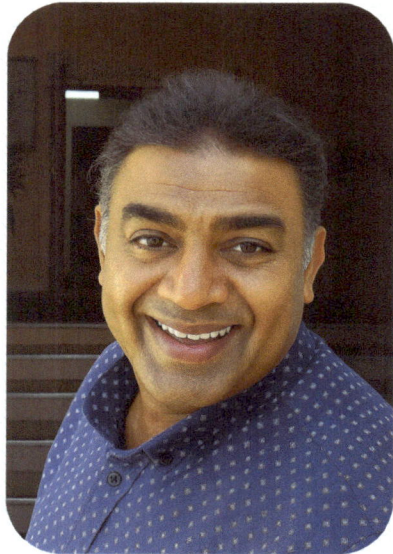

Ready to go out

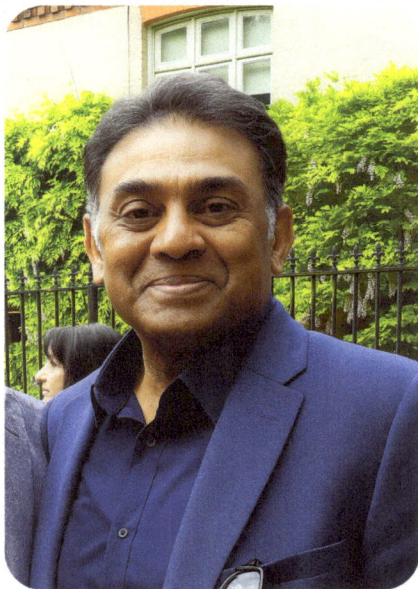

Ready for work

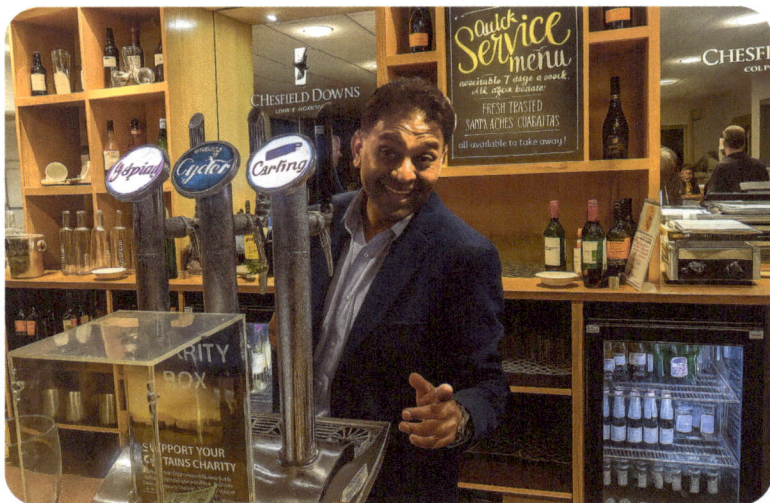

Me behind the bar to serve to my friends

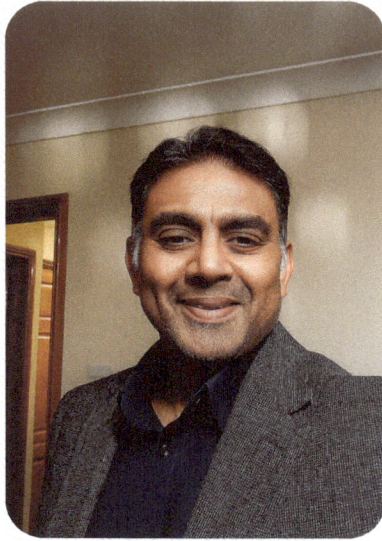

Looking good as ever ready to go out

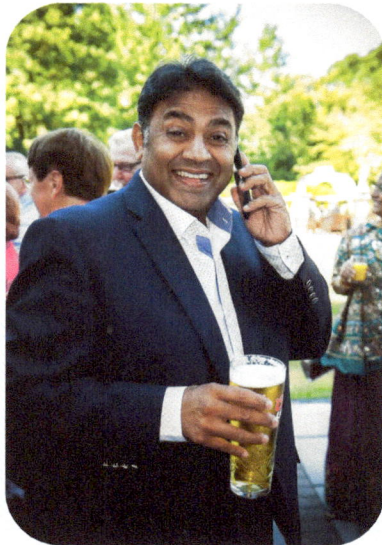

University picture

THE FACES, THE PLACES, THE MEMORIES

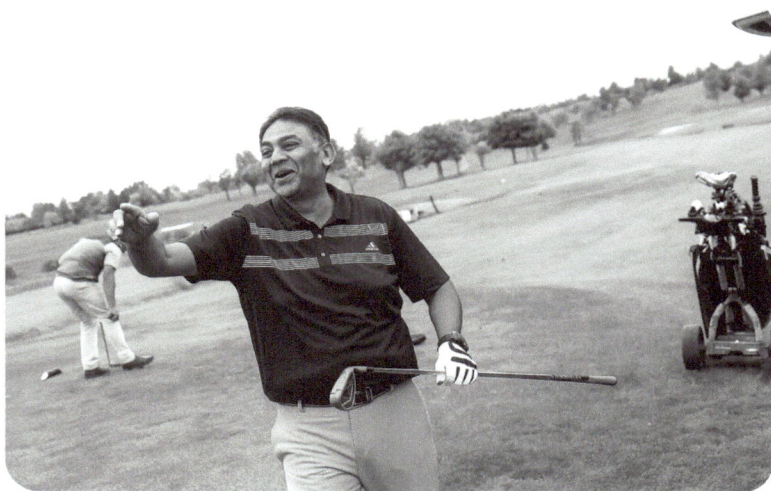

158 Yard drive

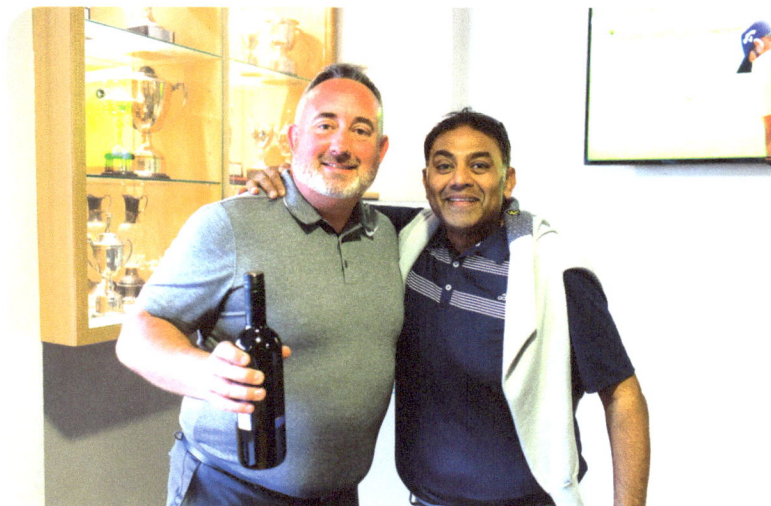

Me congratulating my hinthin brother Simon

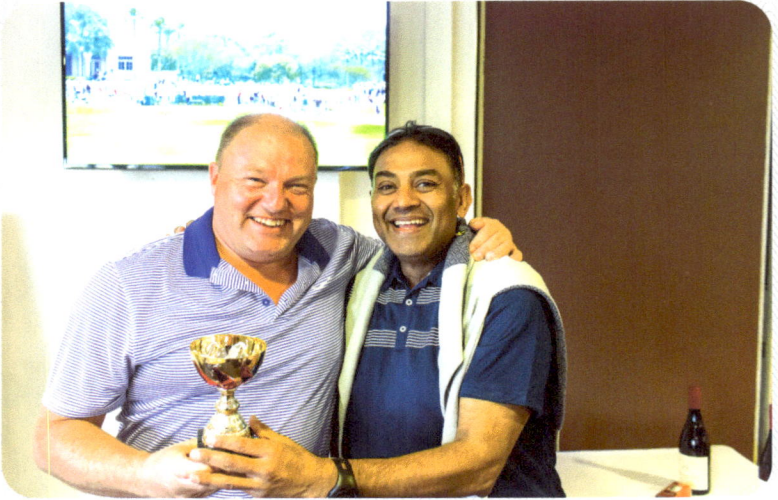

Me giving the Golf Captain a trophy

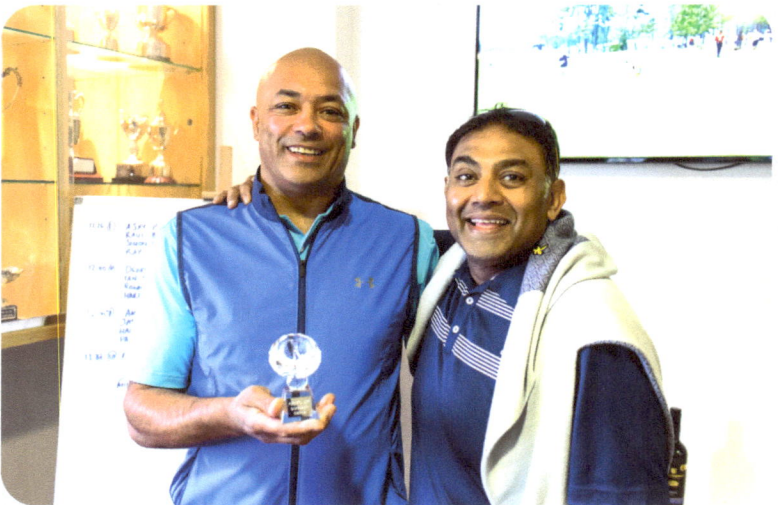

Me presenting Ray the trophy for nearest to the pin

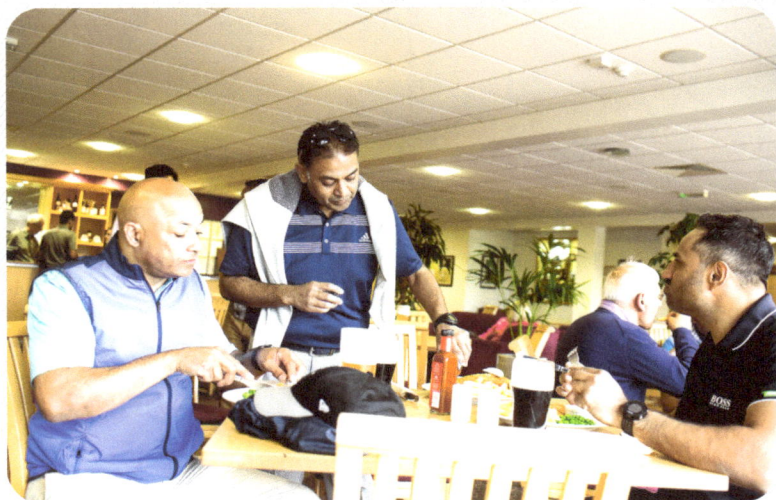

Me pouring wine to my good friend Ravi, showing off my waiter services

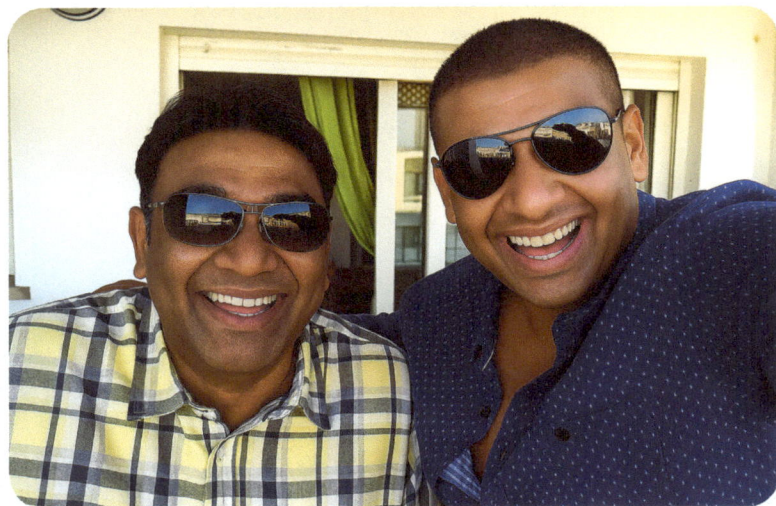

Me with my favrioute nephew Alay

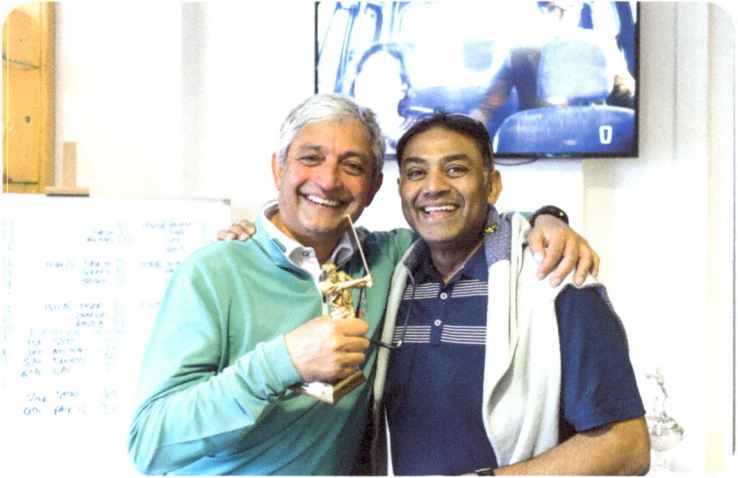

Me with my good friend Jatin

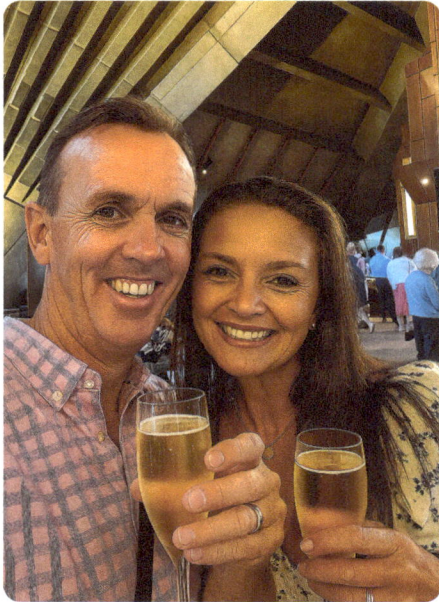

My favrioute work colleague Emma with her husband

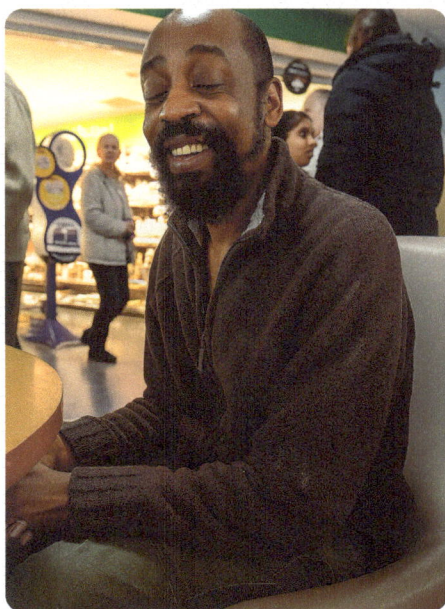

My longest friend for 45 years, Rodney Chandler

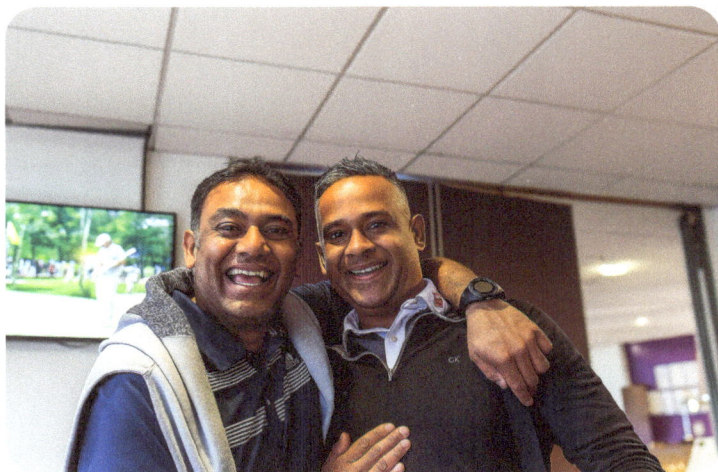

Me and my Mentor Beej

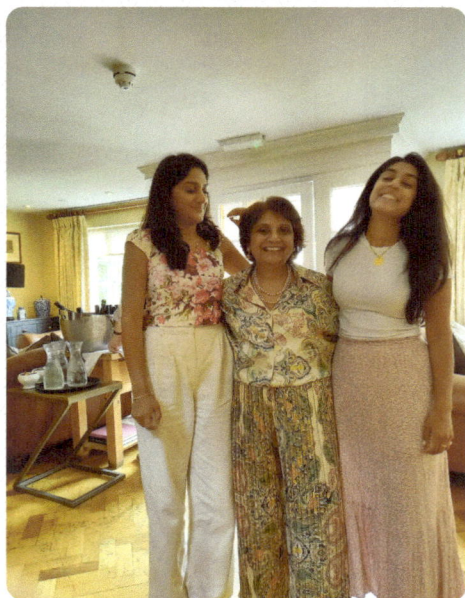

Ladies of the family

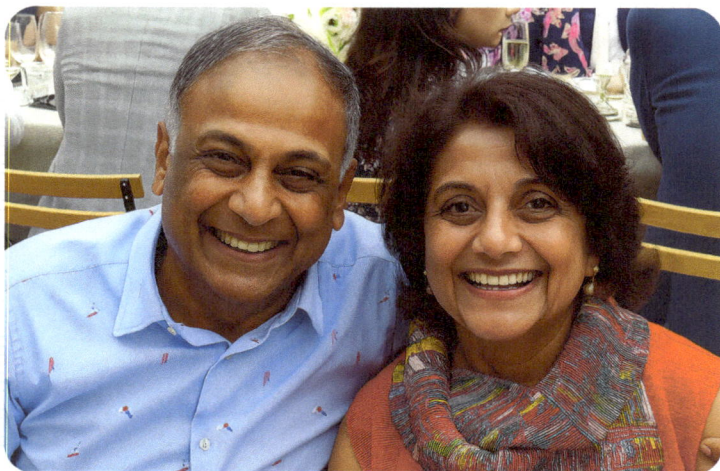

Brother and Sister in law

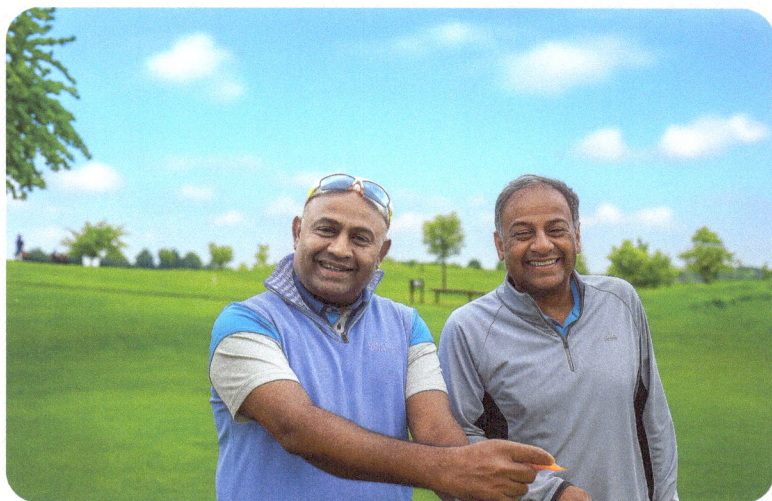

My two brothers – Asit and Amit

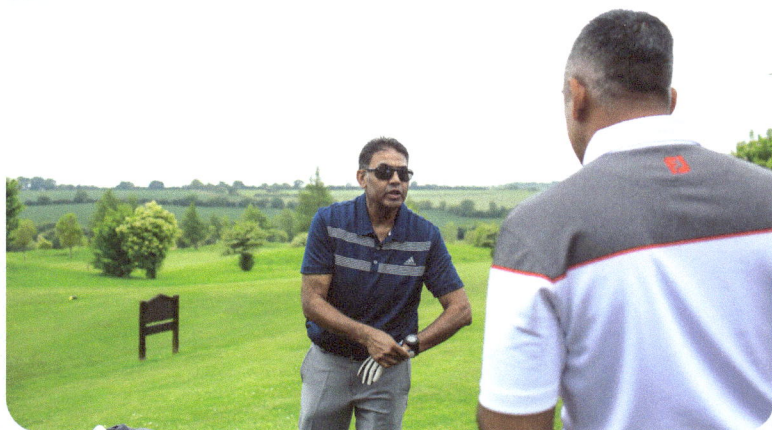

Just letting my Mentor know that he is late again

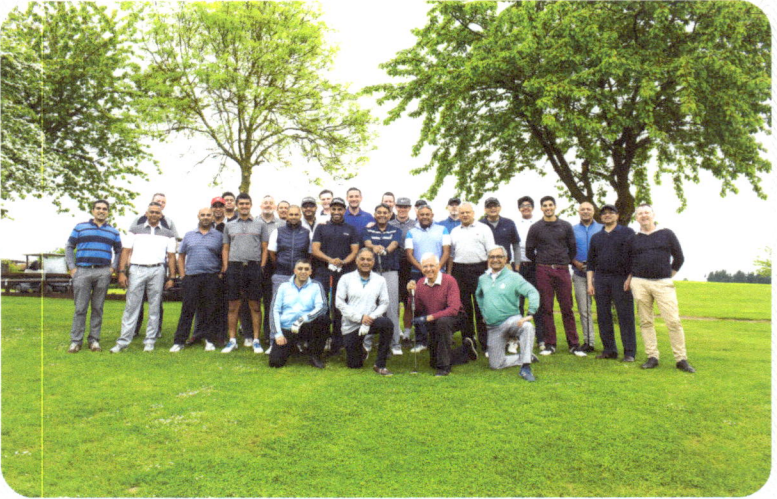

My Birthday golf squad

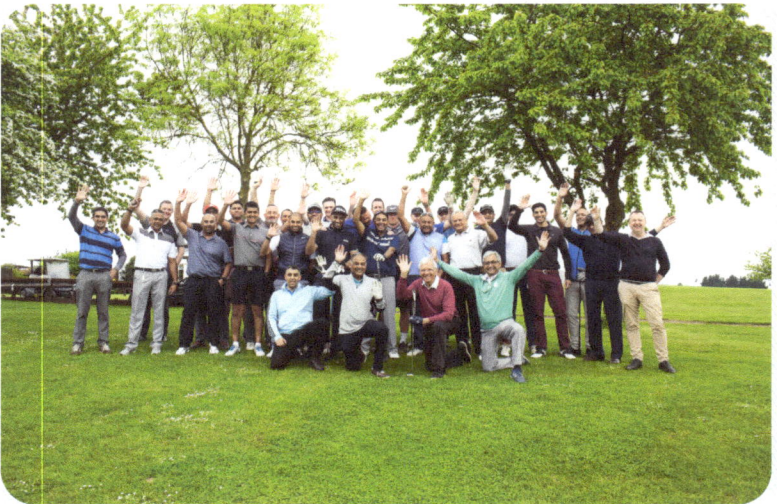

Tee off time

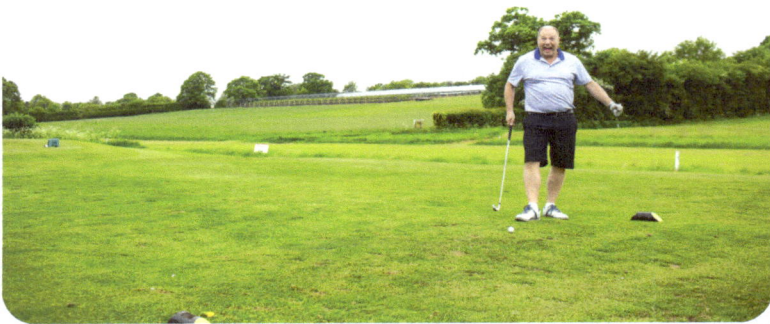

Denchy finally found the tee of green

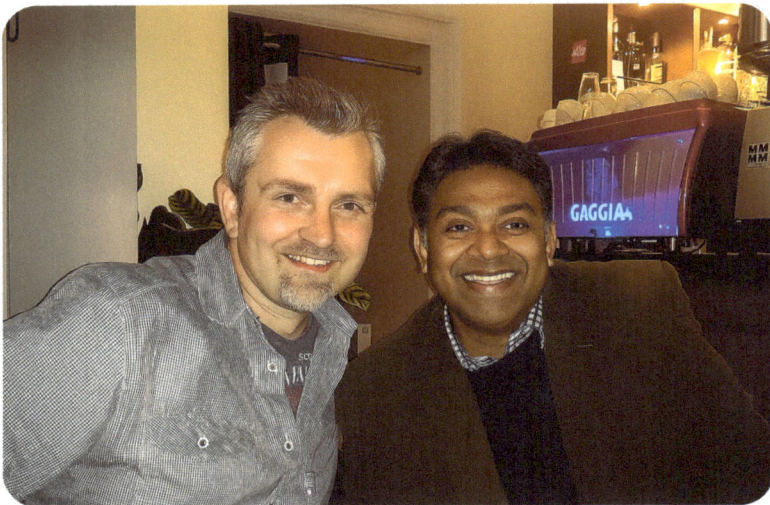

My closest Uni friend Jim

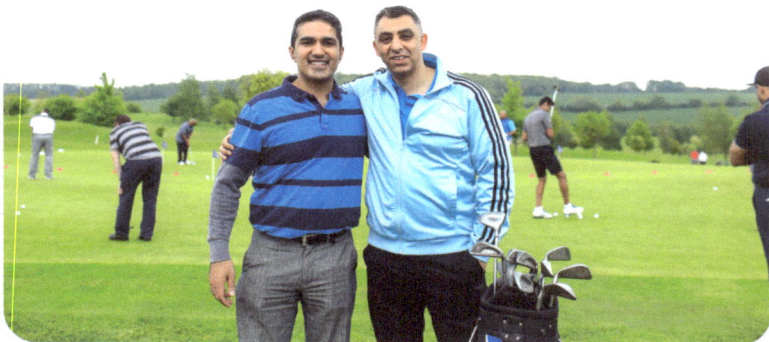

Parthree Boys

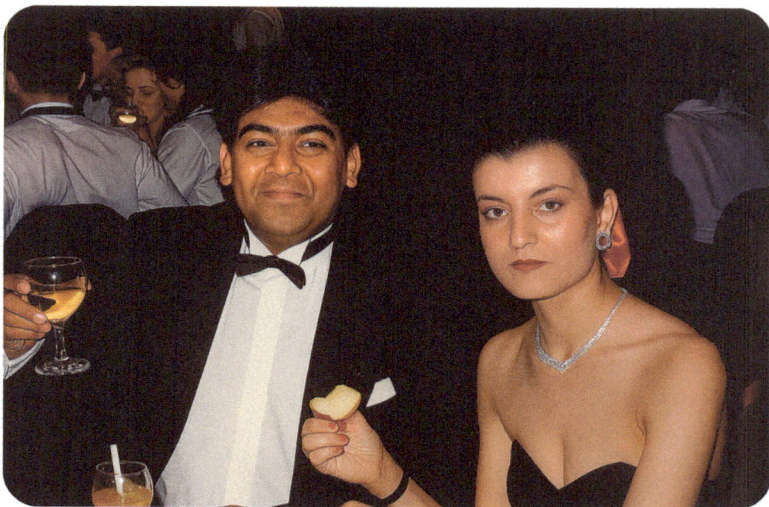

Me with my sweetheart at my first organised dinner dance at Uni

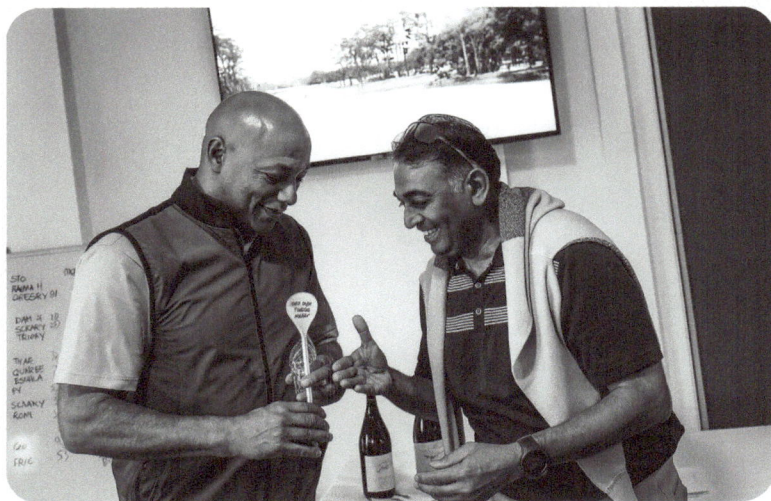

Ray receiving the wooden spoon for coming last

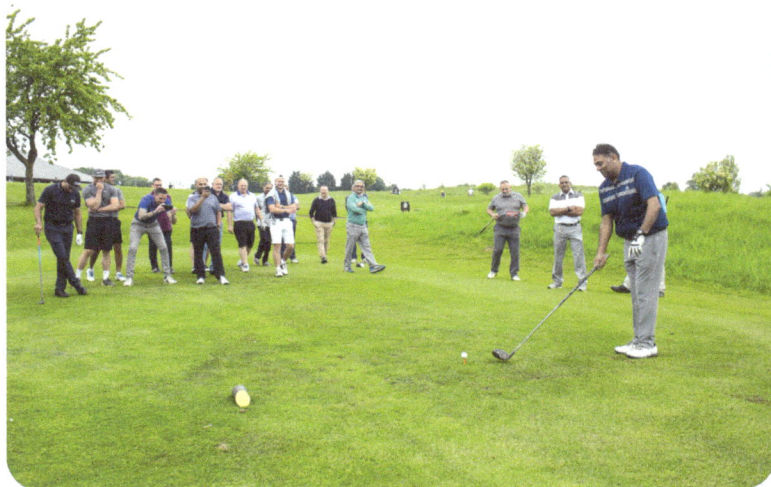

Right hand Golfer

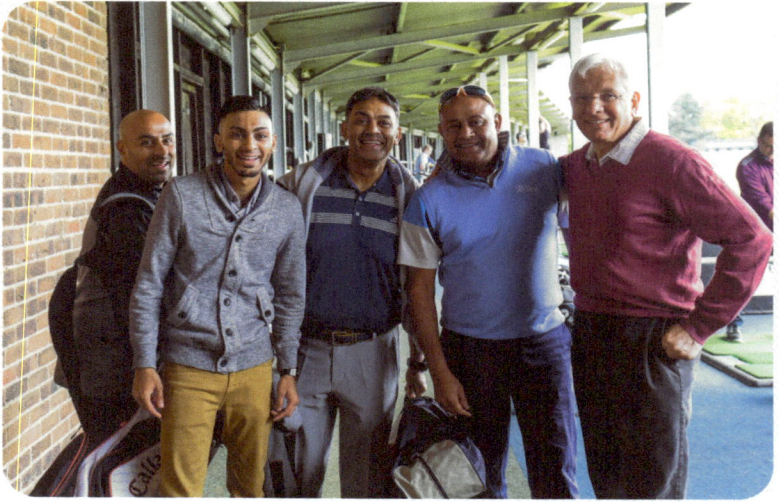

Roaming up at the driving range

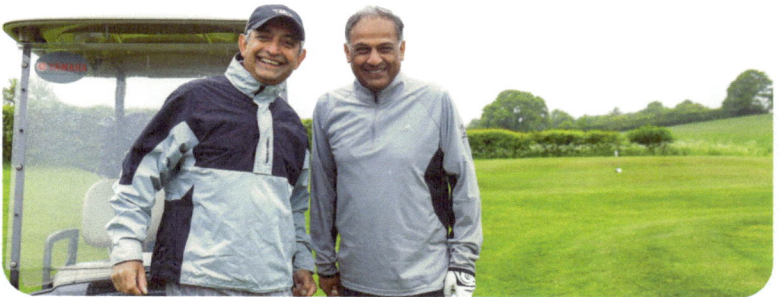

The two beginners enjoying my Birthday Golf day as a practice round

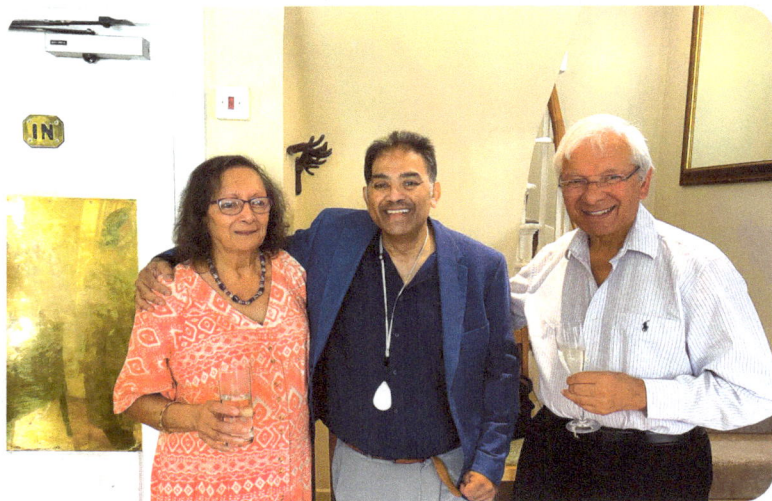

Me with Ramesh Uncle and Illa Aunty

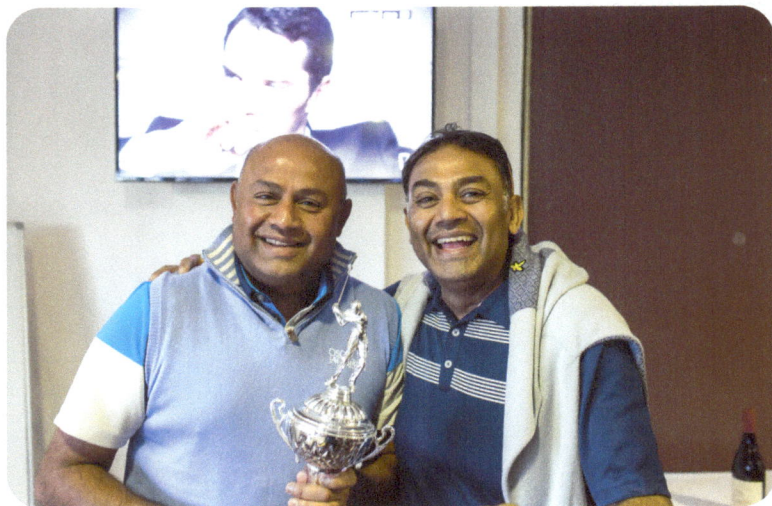

Winner of the day with 40 points

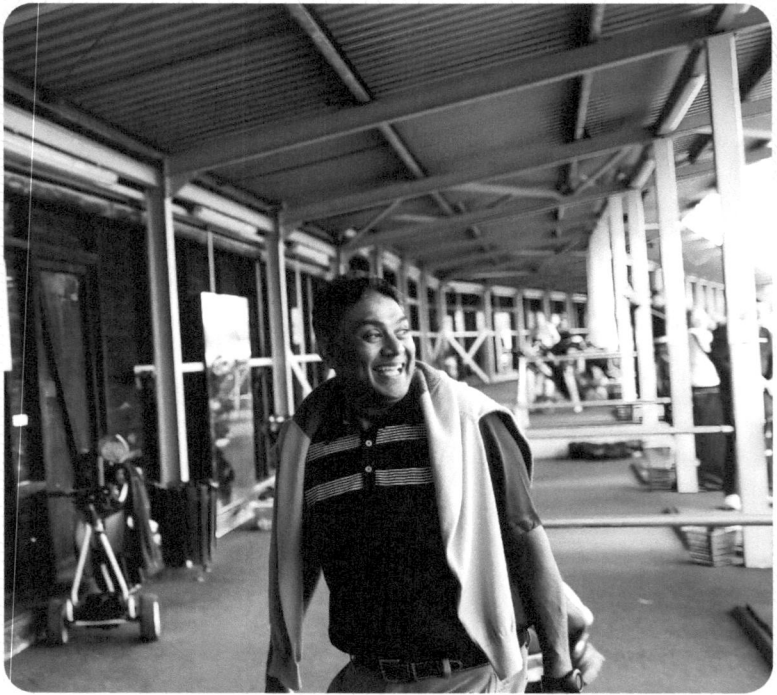

www.ingramcontent.com/pod-product-compliance
Lightning Source LLC
Chambersburg PA
CBHW041308020426
42333CB00001B/11